Get The Mommy Does Yoga DVD!

For Free Prenatal Yoga Videos And Tips, Mommy Inspiration, And All Things Baby Visit Us Anytime At

Mommydoesyoga.com

By Julie Schoen

.

Disclaimer

This book contains general information and is for informational purposes only. You should use proper discretion, and consult with a health care practitioner, before following any of the exercises, techniques, or plans described in this book. The author and publisher expressly disclaim responsibility for any adverse effects that may result from the use or application of the information contained in this book.

CONTENTS:

WELCOME, MOMMIES!

Today I am writing this at 35 weeks pregnant, excitedly awaiting the birth of my second child – a beautiful little girl. The old saying is true, "The days are long but the years are short," as I can hardly believe that my son will be turning two next month. Pregnancy is no different. The nine months pass slowly until all of the sudden you are just weeks away from meeting your little one and you can't believe where time has gone. Being pregnant for a second time has taught me so much. For instance, no two pregnancies are ever the same – ever. My first was easy, no sickness, it felt like there was very little I couldn't do. With my second, feelings of nausea somehow snuck their way into each day for the first four months. I was exhausted, but unable to rest as much as I would have liked thanks to my adorable little toddler who was anxious to show me something new he had discovered or learned. I was violently ill for three days at 16 weeks and at 34 weeks just finished battling a nasty kidney infection.

Pregnancy is, no doubt, an ever changing nine-month journey, no day, no week, ever the same.

But having learned to expect the unexpected this time around I have actually found myself much more relaxed and at ease. I have let go of judgment and comparison, allowing myself to experience the pregnancy rather than try to control it. I have discovered that the most powerful tool we have as expecting mothers is our mindset. If we can strive to find the positive in each struggle, the joy in each pain, the happiness in the changes, we can truly have a blessed experience.

Being pregnant opens one up to a new world, one filled with creativity, expansion, and growth. If you can tap into this realm and awake yourself to the true power you actually hold, you start to notice that nothing is impossible, nothing is too difficult, and that the universe is wholly and completely here to support you.

I have found that practicing yoga while pregnant is not only great for my body, keeping me active while ridding my body of the day's new aches and pains, but it also, maybe even more importantly, strengthens my mind. My practice has evolved from a once ego-filled "I-can-do-that-better" (or, maybe more honestly, "Why-can't-I-do-this-better?") kind of practice to one that embraces exactly where

I'm at on a day-to-day basis. Being pregnant and doing yoga is perhaps the most incredible transformation I have ever experienced as an adult – moving from a life focused on external motivators to one that is centered on all things internal and meaningful.

Whether you have decided to practice yoga for the first time in order to stay healthy and happy while pregnant or have been practicing yoga for years leading up to your pregnancy, you will discover that there is nothing like the experience of prenatal yoga. I urge you to give yourself entirely to the practice each day - it might be a sixty-minute active practice, a ten-minute meditation, or five minutes of stretching before you go to bed. But if you allow yourself to let go and really experience your pregnancy, you will be welcomed into a world of incredible strength and beauty. You will find support on days when you need it most. You will find abundant love on days when you are able to share it with others. You will find everything you need not just for yourself, but for your baby as well.

Congratulations Beautiful Mommies! Much Love To You All,

Julie

THE 5 KEYS TO PRACTICING YOGA WHILE PREGNANT

Prenatal yoga is a wonderful experience for most women, often getting more than they expected from the practice. But for a few, doing yoga while pregnant can be downright frustrating, giving up on the idea altogether after just a class or two. So before you begin practicing, here are five things to keep in mind to help make sure you and your baby get all the good that is there to be had.

1. **Don't Compare Yourself To Anyone, Ever**. Every pregnancy is different just as every body is different. If you come to your practice wanting to be like someone else or look like someone else, you are setting yourself up for disappointment. And it's not because you aren't awesome! In fact, by trying to emulate someone else you are saying to yourself that you're not good enough, when in fact you are. You are a unique, creative, incredible individual. When you are honest and authentic in your life and your practice you discover freedom that leads to joy. Don't miss out on that by focusing on what others are doing or look like. Be true to yourself and your pregnancy.

    "If we mold our practice into some idealized form based on an external standard that is irrelevant to our own destiny, our Yoga practice will only fortify a false sense of self. In this light, always consider your practice in terms of how it can balance and serve the rest of your life. The practice should serve you; you are not a servant to the practice."

    Donna Farhi, Bringing Yoga To Life

2. **Remember It's Okay To Take Care Of Yourself.** Your yoga practice should make you feel amazing, both as you are doing it and when you are done. That's the whole point. For some women, it can be difficult to admit that they need to slow down or that they need to make changes. They are out to prove that being pregnant hasn't changed them – they can still do everything they could do before. And while there is nothing wrong to do much of what you used to love while you are still pregnant, it's important to recognize why you are doing it. Because it feels great? Awesome! Because you want to take a picture of it for Instagram? Maybe something should be reexamined. All in all, just remember that no matter who you are,

pregnancy changes your body and mind dramatically. Embracing those changes, slowing down from time to time, making time for you to feel better, those are all a part of enjoying pregnancy – and those should all be a part of prenatal yoga too.

3. **Prenatal Yoga Is About So Much More Than Exercise.** Yes, prenatal yoga is exercise – and great exercise at that! But there is so much more to it. Practicing prenatal yoga can have a dramatic impact on your mind and spirit. It can help you tap into a state that allows you to think and live in an empirical way, rather than just purely academic. Your mind can shift into a more primal state, tapping into universal forces and experiences that have been present since the beginning of time. Prenatal yoga has the ability to help you prepare for the experience of childbirth, the journey of being a parent, and the millions of changes that will take place starting today. Of course, it doesn't have to. Yoga can just be exercise if that is all you want – and it's still amazing. But if you are looking for more, there is an endless fountain of knowledge waiting to be tapped.

4. **You Are Never Practicing Alone.** You are in an amazing moment of your life, inextricably connected to another human life. Your baby not only feels your movements, but experiences your breath and your thoughts. They see the world how you see it. Even in the womb they are learning as they grow. When you practice prenatal yoga you are making the time to deepen the connection you have with your baby. You are growing the bond you have between mother and child. You are doing so much good! I have found this to be one of the most inspiring revelations of prenatal yoga, and often the main reason why I make it to my mat on days when I feel too busy or simply "not in the mood."

5. **Life Is Ever-Changing And Temporary – Don't Miss A Moment.** Before you know it your baby will be born and this crazy journey of pregnancy will be over. Even if you plan to have another baby (or babies!) in the future, you will never be pregnant exactly like this ever again. Life goes by far too quickly to miss a day. So make it a point to enjoy every day, even those days when you feel horrible, scared, or incredibly overwhelmed. Even on the craziest days, allow yoga to be an escape. A time where you can process what is happening and to take the time to find the joy and excitement, even

if it is only something that seems small. The fact is that those small joys are all that we need to make it through – those are what we remember at the end of our lives. So take a deep breath and enjoy this moment because there will never be another one like it.

PRENATAL MEDITATION TO START AND END YOUR DAY

Go ahead and take a comfortable seat, boosting yourself up onto blankets or a cushion to make sure your hips are higher than your knees. Make the seat as comfortable and easy as possible. You can cross your legs at the shins or ankles, or simply place one foot in front of the other if you need more space. If your knees do not easily reach the floor try sitting on something higher or consider adding pillows or blankets under your thighs so that your legs are supported as you sit. If you feel you would be more comfortable with your back supported against something, like a wall, please do so.

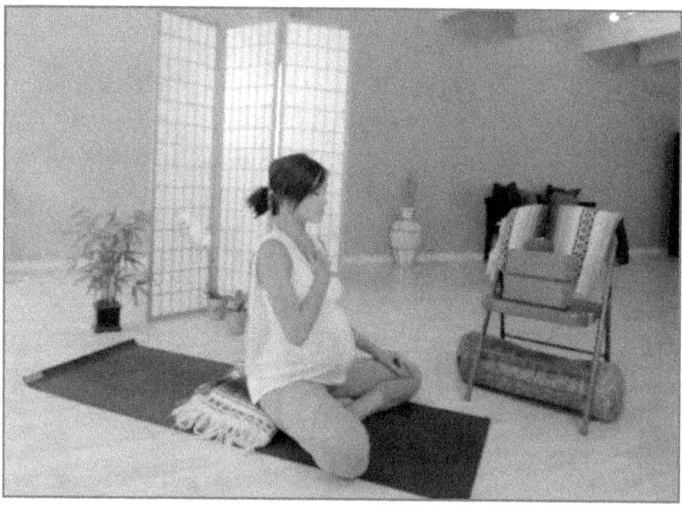

Find both your sit bones, rocking gently from side to side. Settle directly in the middle so that your weight is distributed evenly and you feel spacious and long in your spine. Feel rooted in your seat, as if everything from your waist down is buried under sand. Grow out from the waist, lengthening your side body and creating as much room between your rib bones as possible. As you do this, you make more space for your baby too. Gently draw your front ribs back towards your spine as you relax your shoulders away from your ears, keeping the spine neutral and preventing the sway in the low back that is so common during pregnancy, especially as you and your belly continue to grow.

Soften your throat, relaxing all four sides of your neck as you do. Soften your jaw and your mouth, releasing your tongue away from the roof of your mouth. Keeping your jaw relaxed is so important during pregnancy and can help during labor and delivery as well. Remind yourself to soften your jaw as much as possible throughout your practice and your day. Soften the area around your eyes, releasing your gaze to the center of your forehead, just between the eyebrows – your third eye.

Allow your hands to rest naturally on your knees or thighs, palms up or down, whichever is more comfortable today. Allow the elbows to rest under your shoulders and your hands and fingers to relax.

Begin to notice your breath, doing your best to be a quiet observer, trying not to change or alter anything about it.

What does your breath sound like?

What does your breath feel like?

No judgment – just observe.

Notice the cool air at the base of your nose at the beginning of each inhalation. Notice the warm air at the end of each exhalation. Cool air enters as you inhale, warm air leaves as you exhale. Remind yourself that each breath you take – your baby feels. You are wonderfully and incredibly connected at this moment. As you draw energy in through your breath you are feeding, growing, and nourishing your little one.

Imagine that with each breath you take you are not just taking in air, but light. See the light as it enters through your nose, travels down your throat, and enters at the center of your heart.

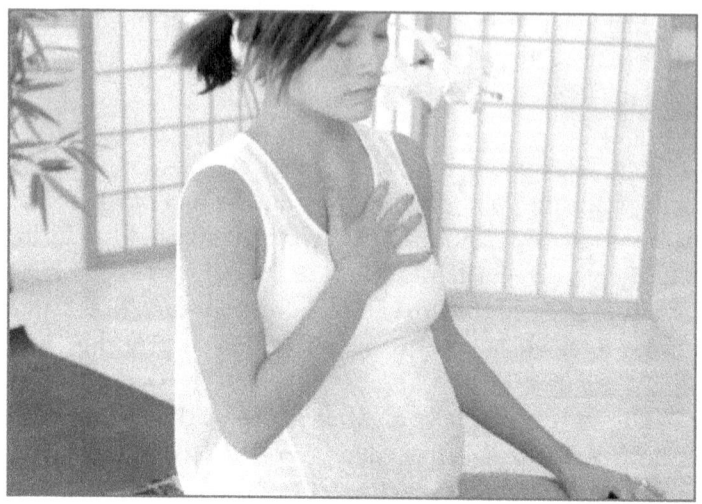

See your heart receiving this light with each inhale and expanding and growing with light on each exhale. As your heart grows you are reminded that love is abundant. There is always more than enough. Love grows. Love is created. Pregnancy itself is all about growth and creation. Creative forces not only create a beautiful new human life, but they change how you see, how you think, how you feel. These forces also create love. Love without boundaries. Love without limits. Love without end. Love like you have never known before.

With each breath remind yourself that:

You are loved. You are taken care of. You have everything you need.

You are loved. You are taken care of. You have everything you need.

Imagine the breath and light. See them now not just stopping at your heart, but traveling down, through your womb, and into your little one. See your baby's heart receiving the light and expanding with love and gratitude just as yours is.

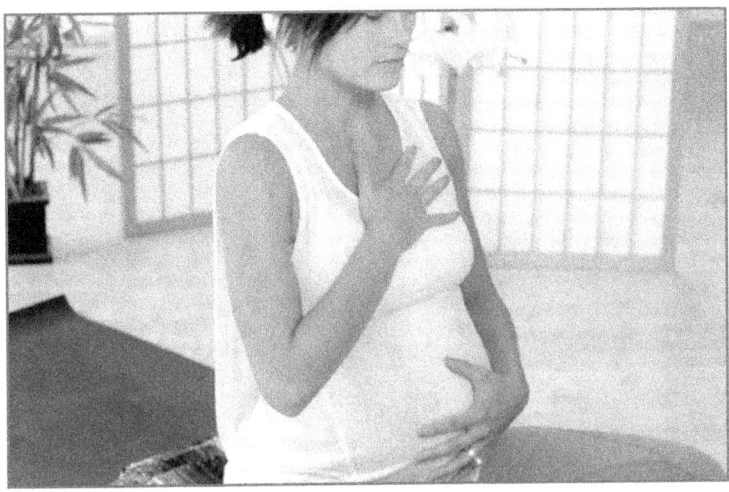

Your baby can feel your thoughts, so with each breath you take send a message:

I love you. I will take care of you. I am all that you need.

I love you. I will take care of you. I am all that you need.

From the earth, visualize a radiant green light growing, enveloping you and your baby in a place of love and safety. Let this light wrap you up like a cocoon, offering support, offering protection. In this green light you and your baby share breath, share thoughts, share movements, share love.

With each breath be reminded that:

You are both loved. You are both taken care of. You both have everything you need.

You are both loved. You are both taken care of. You both have everything you need.

MOMMY DOES YOGA ACTIVE POSES

These poses can be practiced in order from beginning to end or you can simply choose a handful to practice, focusing on one thing in particular, whether it's your breath, opening your shoulders, or strengthening your legs. As you practice feel free to hold each pose for as long as it feels good. If you start to feel out of breath or tired, take rest. Remember that each day will be different so don't ever feel like you have to do exactly what you did before. Listen to your body, listen to your baby, and take care!

1. Seated Spinal Circles

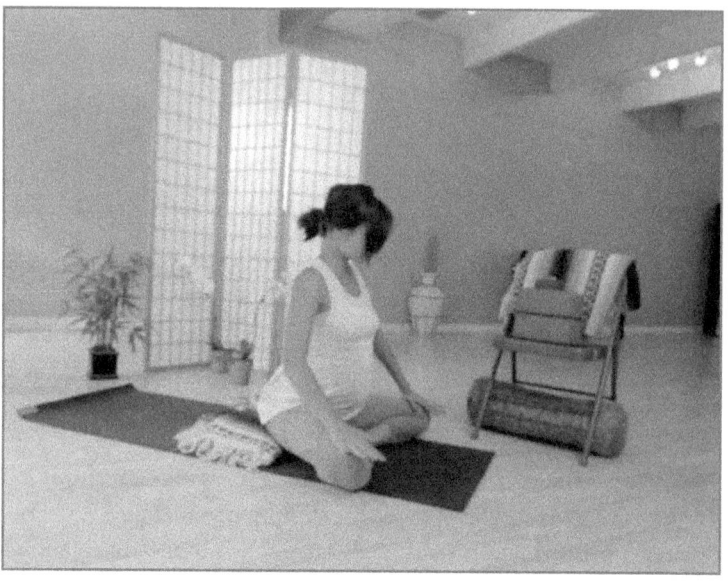

From a comfortable seat, propped up on blankets or a cushion to ensure your hips are higher than your knees. Place your hands on your thighs or the floor in front of you, being mindful that whatever position you choose you are providing your baby with plenty of room. With an inhalation begin to arch your back, rocking the weight forward on your pelvis. Draw the side ribs to the right, slightly lifting the right shoulder towards the ear. On the exhalation round the back, tipping the weight back onto your pelvis and drawing the chin towards the chest slightly. Continue the movement by moving the side ribs to the left, slightly lifting the left shoulder towards the ear.

With your next inhalation start the cycle again, moving as fast or as slow as feels good. Be sure to keep your jaw and face relaxed as you move, being as fluid as possible. After 5 to 10 rounds one direction, change directions.

2. Marjaryasana – Bitilasana

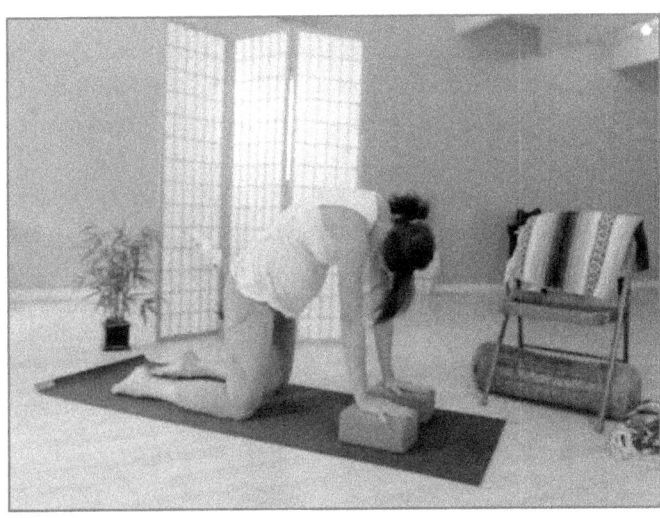

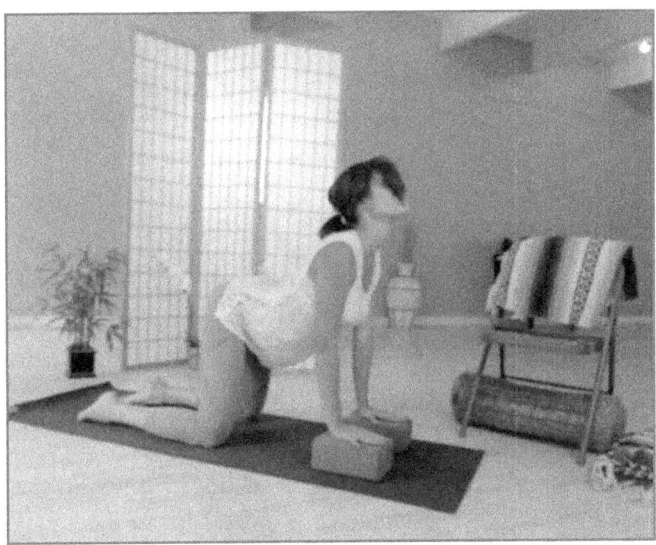

Come to all fours, hands shoulder-width apart or wider and knees and feet hip-width apart or wider. If you are farther along in your pregnancy, consider placing your hands on blocks or elevating them to take some of the weight off of your wrists. Spread your fingers wide and press down through all ten toenails. Take a deep breath through your nose. As you exhale, press your hands and tops of the feet into the mat, like you are pressing them away from you. Energize your arms and round your back, drawing the chin towards the chest. With your next inhalation, draw the shoulder blades towards each other, lifting the chest and chin forward and up. Continue moving from cat pose to cow pose, using the breath as a guide for pace. Do 5 to 10 rounds total.

When practicing these poses prenatal, it's a good idea to focus more on the movement in the upper back than emphasizing the work in the pelvis as is traditionally taught in these poses. Pregnant women want to be mindful not to overstretch or compress the abdominal area, especially as baby grows and space is limited.

3. **Flying Dog,** *variation*

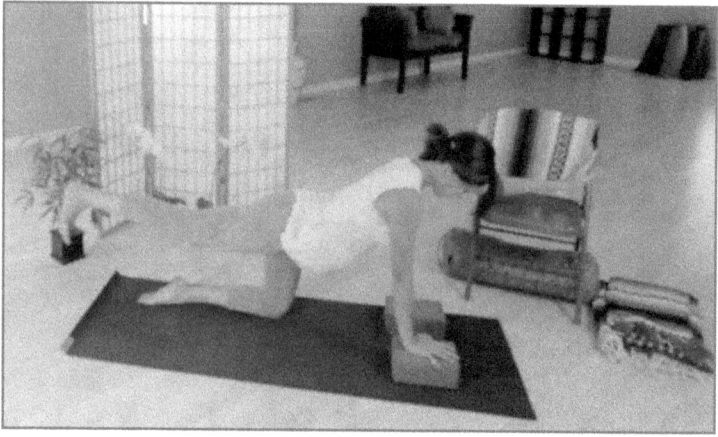

From all fours, lift the right knee off the mat, extending the leg straight so that it is level with the floor. Circle the ankle both directions, encouraging blood flow and reducing swelling in the joint. If possible, at the same time lift the left hand off the mat, extending the arm straight so that it is also level with the floor. Begin to circle the wrist in both directions. Take 4 to 5 breaths in this position before switching sides.

If it feels too unstable to lift both the leg and the opposite arm at the same time, lift just the leg first and then the arm.

The core should feel slightly engaged as you do this, like you are giving your baby a hug, but not overly strained at any point.

4. **Marjaryasana – Bitilasana (Cat – Cow Pose), *variation***

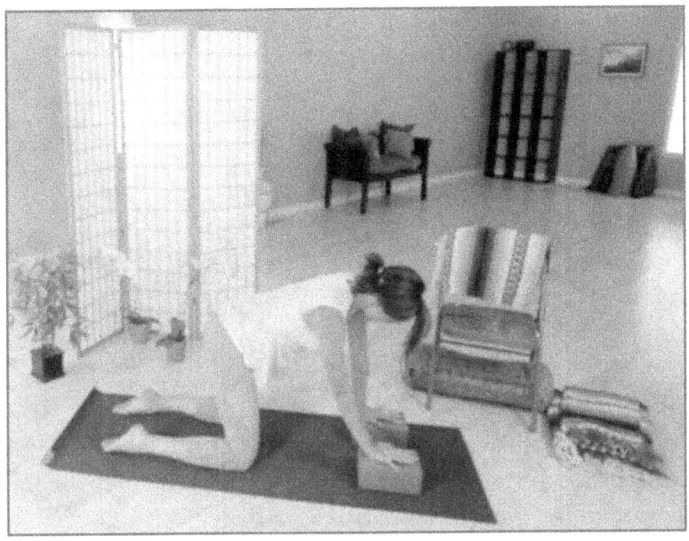

Staying on all fours, return your hands and knees to the ground. Make sure your fingers are spread wide and you are using blocks under your hands if you feel any discomfort in your wrists in this position. Adding on to the Cat-Cow pose done previously, imagine you are inside a glass bottle. The goal is to touch all four sides of the bottle as you move through the poses.

As you inhale, arch the back and open the chest, moving your belly down towards the ground. Continuing on the inhalation, move your hips to the right. As you exhale, round your back and press the area between the shoulders up towards the ceiling and bringing your chin towards your chest. On the same breath, move your hips to the left. Start the cycle again with your next inhalation.

Repeat the cylindrical motion 4 to 5 times in one direction before switching directions. Stay mindful of the breath as you move and try to keep your movements as fluid and smooth as possible.

5. Balasana (Child's Pose)

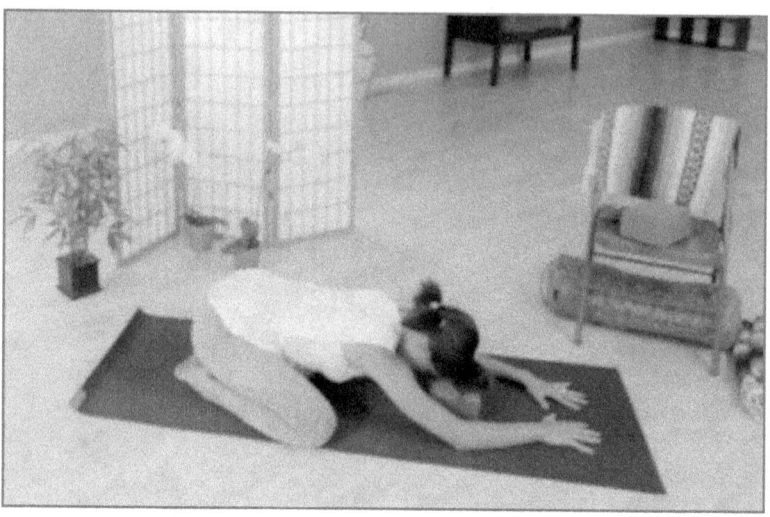

From all fours, take your knees wide and bring your feet together, big toes touching. The further along you are in your pregnancy the wider your knees will need to be to accommodate your growing baby. Begin to bring your hips back towards your heels. Lengthen your spine and place the forehead down on the ground.

If you are in your third trimester or if placing your head on the ground causes your hips to move away from your heels, elevate your head by placing a block, pillow or bolster under your forehead.

Stretch your arms forward, palms facing down and elbows bending slightly. Release your tongue from the roof of your mouth and relax the jaw and face. Take several deep breaths here.

This pose is very restful and should be taken anytime you feel tired or out of breath as you practice. It is also a great pose to take anytime throughout the day, as it is extremely soothing to the nervous system. Some pregnant women also find relief from nausea and morning sickness in this asana.

6. **Tadasana with Urdhva Hastasana (Mountain Pose with Upward Salute)**

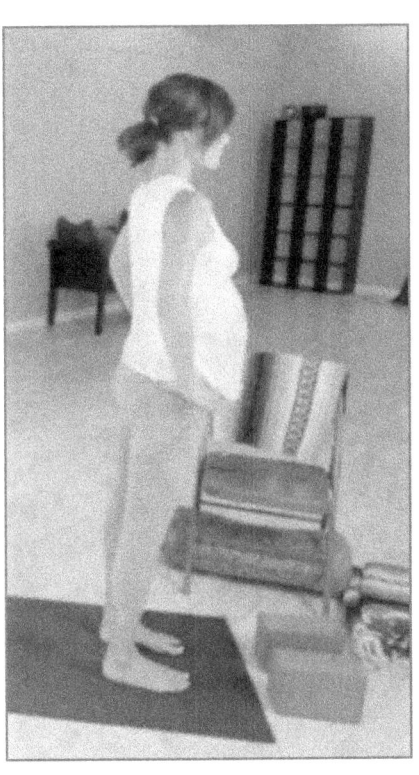
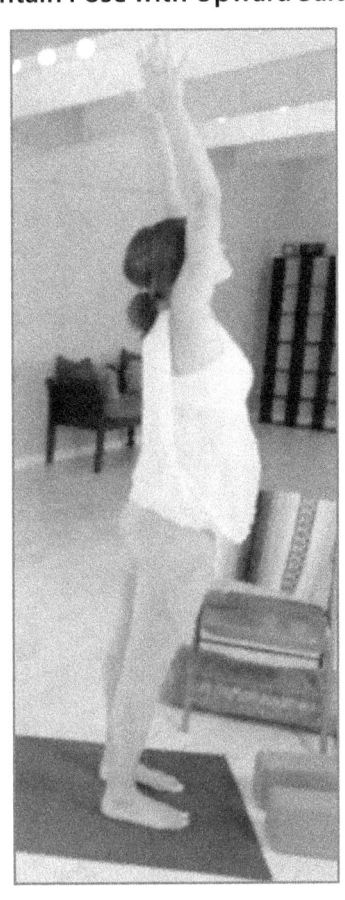

Come to stand at the top of your mat with feet at least hip-width apart. The wider your stance the more stable and supported you will feel as your belly grows. Press firmly through all four corners of your feet, spreading your toes and lifting up through the center of the arches of the feet. Lengthen through all four sides of the ankles. Engage the quadriceps muscles of the thighs, lifting the kneecaps without locking the knees. Gently rotate your upper inner thighs back to create a sense of broadening in the low back. Draw your tailbone down towards your heels as you simultaneously lift your front hipbones up. Soften your front ribs to prevent dramatic sway in your low back. Release the shoulders away from your ears. Draw the chin back slightly to align your total spine.

As you breathe in this position imagine the breath not only expanding the chest front to back, but also side to side.

Keeping this position intact, from Mountain Pose began to add the Upward Salute by drawing your arms out to the side and reaching the arms up over your head on an inhalation. As you exhale, release the hands back down by your sides or in prayer position at your heart center. Continue moving the arms with the breath, repeating 5 to 10 times.

7. **Uttanasana (Standing Forward Bend),** *variation*

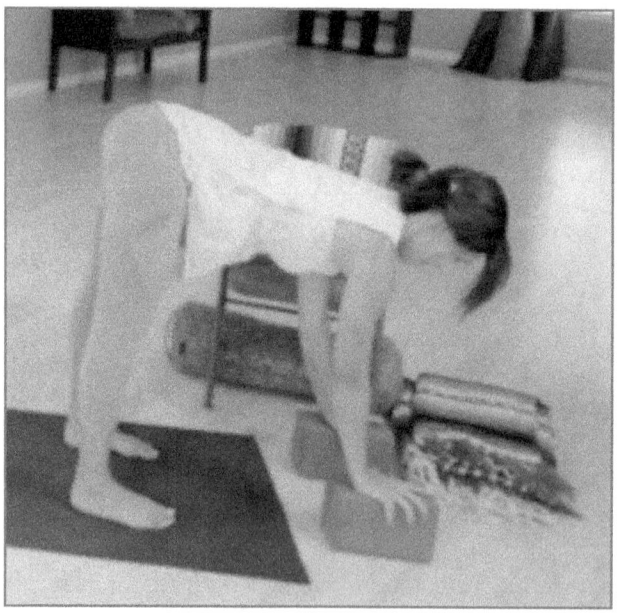

From Mountain Pose, begin to hinge forward from your hips, stopping the moment the belly begins to feel compressed. As the belly grows, the back will become more parallel with the floor, rather than perpendicular, which is how the pose is traditionally done. For most women, blocks will be needed under the hands in order to maintain proper alignment without any compression.

Although you may not be folding as deep as you used to, you can still get a great stretch for the backs of the legs as well as a sublime release for the low back. Focus on lengthening through the spine, keeping the hips pinned back so that they are right over the ankles. Keep the legs engaged in the same manner you did in Mountain Pose, continuing to draw the upper inner thighs back. Draw the chin slightly to the chest so that the neck is not craning forward and take several deep breaths.

8. **Anjaneyasana (Low Lunge)**

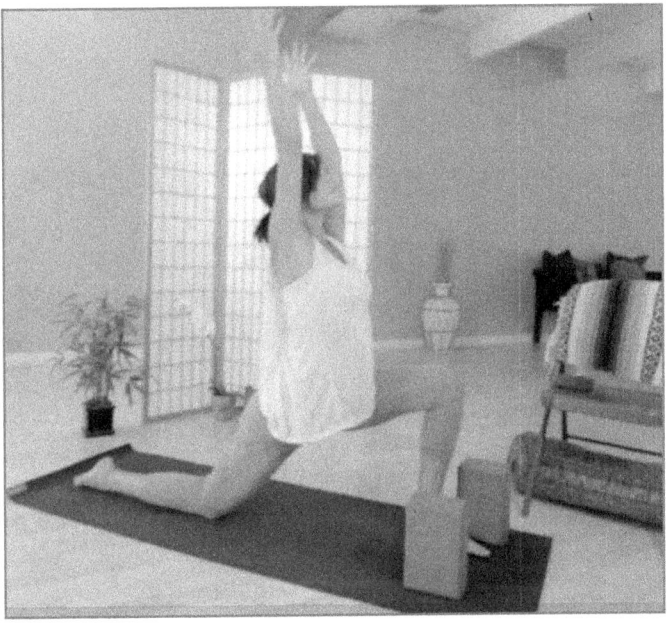

From the previous pose, Uttanasana, carefully step the right foot back, using the blocks as necessary for support. Place the right knee down on the mat, pointing the right toes so that the top of the foot is also on the mat. Make sure your left knee is directly over the ankle. Place your hands on your left thigh to encourage the thighbone to move down as you lift the left hipbone away from the thigh.

As you inhale, sweep the arms up and over your head, spreading the fingers and keeping the shoulders relaxed. Shift your gaze up slightly. You should feel a nice stretch in the right hip and the front of the right leg, but it should never at any time feel like there is any pulling taking place. If you feel like you are overstretching, shift your weight back more or take a shorter stance.

To feel supported and balanced in this pose, isometrically draw the left heel back, as if you were dragging the front of the mat back, while simultaneously pressing the right knee forward. This action should not only feel stabilizing, but also freeing for the pelvis and low back. Hold this pose for 5 to 6 breaths.

As you exhale, place your hands on the ground inside your left leg and return to all fours. From all fours step your right foot forward and repeat the pose on the other side.

9. Plank Pose

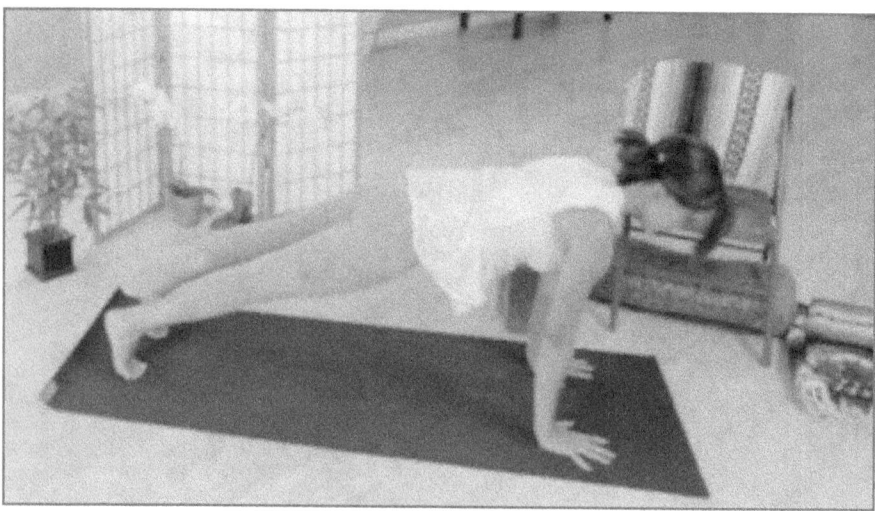

From all fours, lift your knees off the ground. Work to get your body in one parallel line with the floor. Your feet should remain hip-width apart and your hands under your shoulders – your arms acting like two strong pillars. Bring your gaze just off the front of your mat so that the back of your neck stays elongated. Draw your tailbone down as you lift your hipbones up. Spread through the fingers to support your wrists.

Hold this pose for as long as is comfortable, dropping the knees down whenever you need to rest. Try to stay in the pose for a total of 8 to 10 breaths. Once again you should feel the core engaging slightly, giving your baby a hug without overly constricting the space in the abdomen.

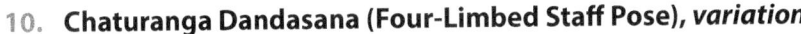

10. Chaturanga Dandasana (Four-Limbed Staff Pose), *variation*

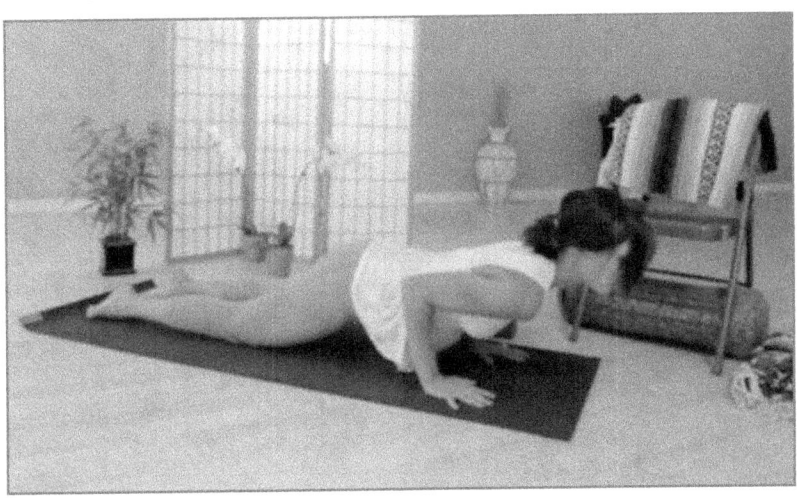

From Plank Pose, set your knees on the ground. Lengthen the spine and shift your weight forward slightly. Looking forward, begin to bend the elbows, keeping the close, if not touching, to your side body. Lower down only as far as your belly will let you, making sure the arms stop at a 90-degree position, with the shoulders in line with the elbows and the elbows directly above the wrists. You can keep the feet hip-width apart as you practice this pose.

Depending on how far along you are, you may still practice this pose with the knees of the ground. Remember, however, that this pose is very difficult and that there is no need to push yourself here during pregnancy. You will have plenty of time for all of the full-on Chaturangas you want after you have your baby, so don't feel bad about resting or modifying when necessary.

11. Urdhva Mukha Svanasana (Upward Facing Dog Pose), *variation*

From your modified Chaturanga Dandasana, press into the palms of your hands and begin to straighten the arms, keeping your knees and tops of the thighs down on the mat. Lift the heart up towards the ceiling while shifting your gaze up as well. Try to draw the shoulders back to prevent them from collapsing forward. Drawing the bottom tips of the shoulder blades down the back can help keep the shoulders from collapsing as well.

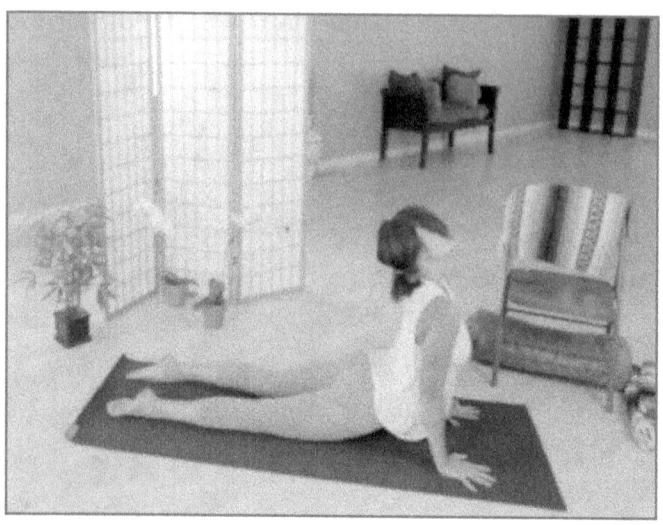

Keeping your knees down help to prevent straining in this pose while pregnant while also making the backbend milder, ensuring that you do not overstretch the front of the body, especially the abdomen.

Traditionally this pose is just held for one breath as you flow into the next pose, but if you find that it feels wonderful (which many pregnant women do), don't hesitate to stay here for as long as you'd like!

12. Adho Mukha Svanasana (Downward Facing Dog)

From the modified Upward Facing Dog Pose, return to all fours. Move the hands out from under the shoulders a few inches and spread the fingers wide, making sure that the index fingers are parallel with the long edges of the mat. Your hands should be at least shoulder-width apart.

Lift your knees off the mat, straightening the legs and pressing back into your heels. Don't worry if your heels are not touching the mat. Make sure your feet are at least hip-width apart.

This pose can feel great for the back as it shifts so much of the weight that settles into the pelvis and low back. Try pressing through your hands more and lifting out of the shoulder sockets to feel even more elongation in the spine. To create more space in the low back, rotate your upper inner thighs back and up towards the ceiling. Engage the quadriceps muscles of the thighs and move the thighbones back so that your legs begin to take some of the weight off your hands and wrists.

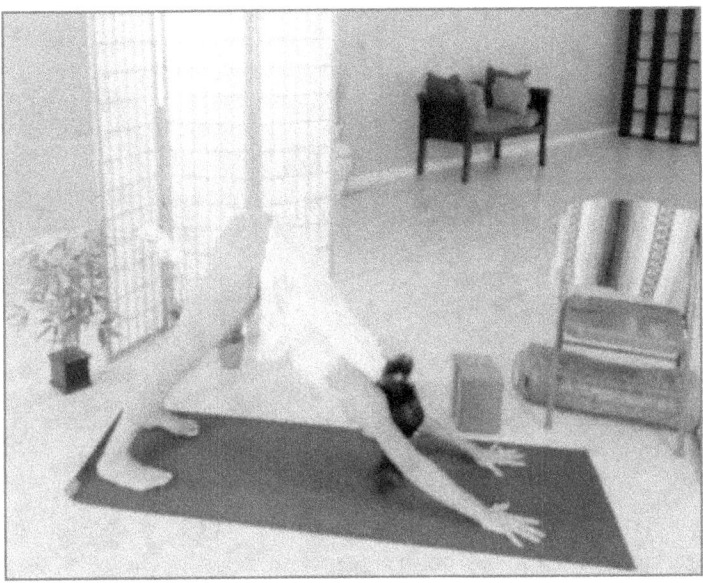

Hold this pose for several breaths (up to 10). When you feel like you need a break, drop the knees down to the floor. You can actually create much of the same effect of this pose in the spine with the knees down simply by reaching the arms forward and keeping the hips over the knees (often this pose is called "Puppy Pose").

13. **High Lunge,** *variation* **– (Insert High Lunge Image)**
From Downward Facing Dog or all fours, carefully step the right foot forward, placing the ankle directly under the knee. Curl the toes of your left foot under and begin to lift the knee off the mat. If this does not feel stable, feel free to repeat Low Lunge with the back knee down. During pregnancy, don't feel like you need to straighten the back leg completely, as it can feel great to keep a small bend in the knee. With an inhalation, sweep the arms up towards the ceiling, palms facing each other and fingers spreading wide. Be mindful not to overarch the back as you practice this pose. Remember to draw the front ribs down and keep the tailbone tucking under.

Return to all fours and repeat on the other side.

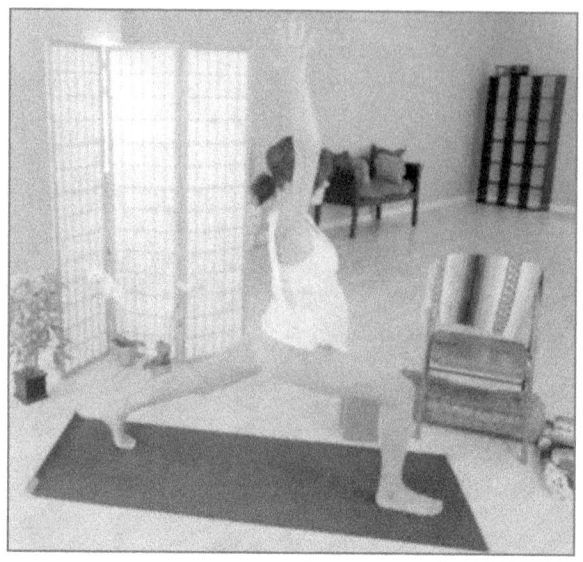

As a variation, you can draw your hands behind you rather than up and interlace your fingers behind your back. This is a great way to open the chest and shoulders, two areas that tend to get very tight as they are pulled forward during pregnancy. With the hands interlaced, press back through the knuckles and begin to lift the hands up towards the ceiling to deepen the stretch.

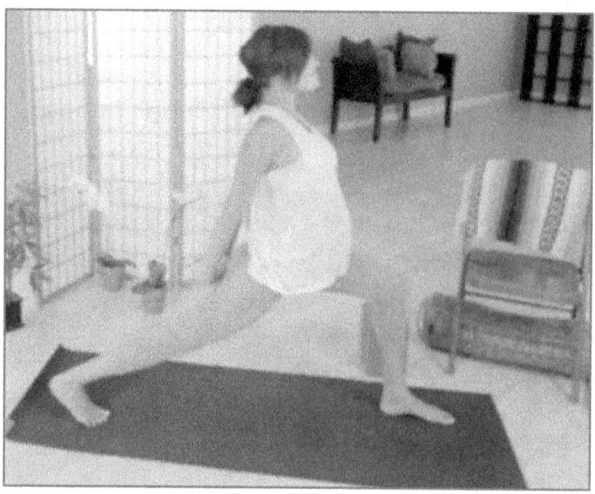

14. **Virabhadrasana II (Warrior II Pose)**

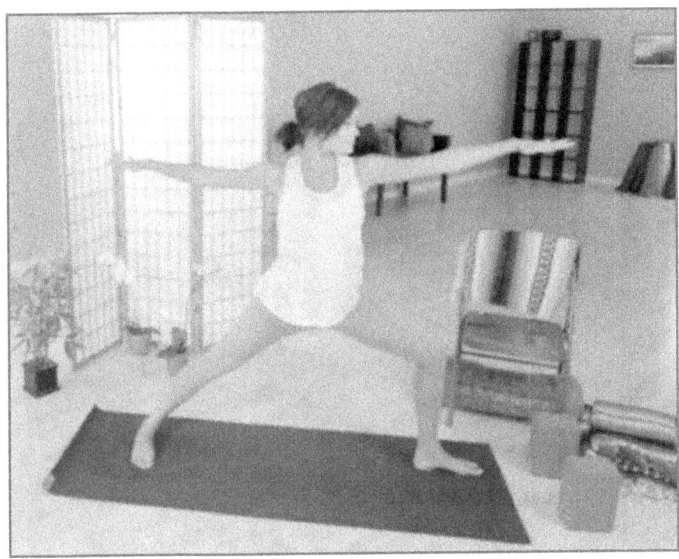

Begin from a standing position at the top of your mat and then carefully step back with your right foot. Bend your left knee as much as is comfortable, making sure the knee stays over the ankle and you don't feel any pulling in the left hip or pressure in the pubic area. If you do, shorten your stance or try not bending your knee so much. Angle your back right foot so that the toes are at a 45-degree angle from the top of your mat. Your heels should be in line with each other or wider, especially if you are in your third trimester or are feeling unstable.

Extend the arms, bringing the backs of the arms level with the ground, palms facing down. Engage your triceps muscles by pulling the backs of the arms up towards the arm bone. Relax your shoulders and your face while spreading your toes to ensure you are not gripping through the feet.

Take 4 to 5 breaths in this pose before turning to the back of your mat and repeating on the other side.

15. **Virabhadrasana II (Warrior II Pose), *variation***

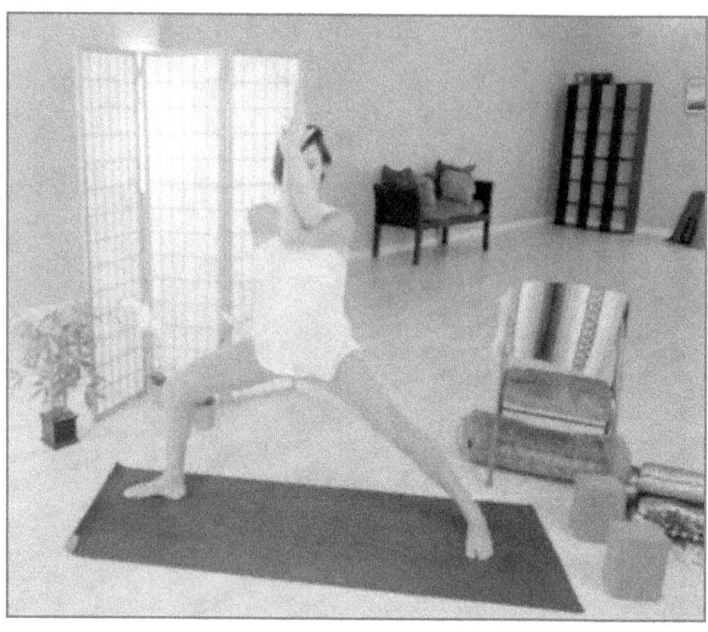

As a variation to the Warrior II Pose described above, you can add a stretch for your shoulders and upper back by changing the position of your arms. With the arms extended as in Warrior II, cross one arm under the other at the elbows. Take the bottom arm and see if you can cross that wrist over the other, coming into what is known in yoga as *Garuda* (Eagle) arms. If possible bring the palms of the hands together.

Turn your torso so that you are facing the side of your mat. With an inhalation, raise the backs of the arms so that they are level with the ground. As you exhale, squeeze the elbows and wrists together to deepen the stretch. Hold this pose for 4 to 5 breaths before releasing the arms and repeating on the other side.

16. **Utthita Trikonasana (Extended Triangle Pose)**

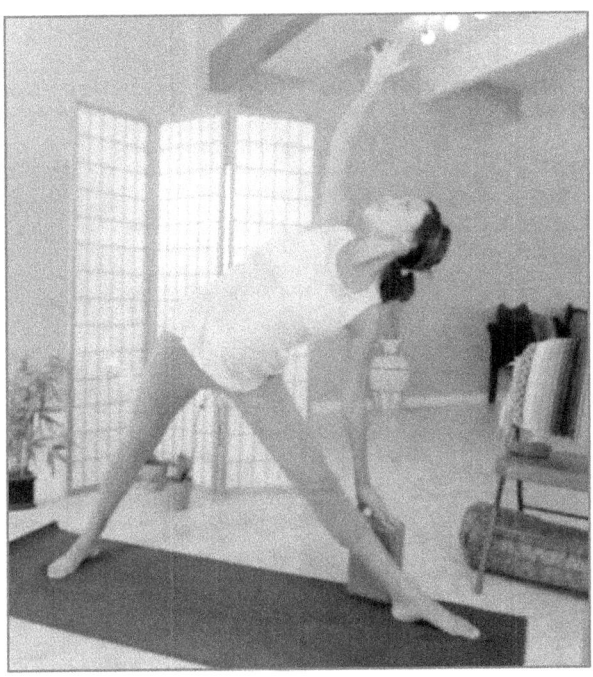

With a block nearby on your left side, step the right foot back from the top of the mat. Your back toes should be at a 45-degree angle from the top of the mat and your front toes pointing straight forward. With both legs straight, begin to hinge from the left hip, sliding your left hand down the front leg, placing it either on the shin or block. Extend your right arm up towards the ceiling, working to get two arms in one line. If it is comfortable for your neck, bring your gaze to your extended hand.

The goal in this pose is to keep the side body in one line. For most people, especially pregnant women, the tendency is to allow the body to lean forward, taking the side body out of a straight line. To prevent this from happening, don't try to get the bottom arm down as far as possible. Use a block or your leg to create space through the spine and ribs. Imagine you are trying to lean your entire back body against a wall behind you. Or, think about keeping the ankle, knee, hip, shoulder, and ear on the side of the body that is stretching all in one line.

Hold this pose for 5 to 6 breaths before slowly bringing yourself up and repeating on the other side.

17. **Utthita Parsvakonasana (Extended Side Angle),** *variation*

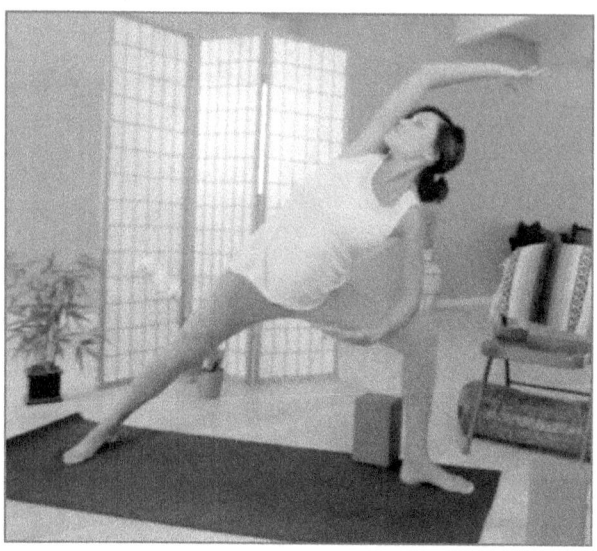

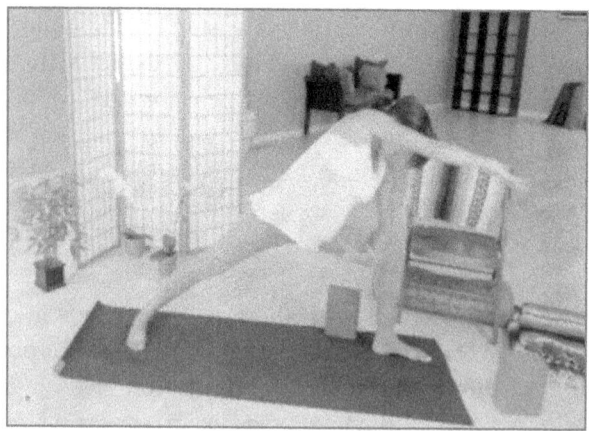

Standing at the top of your mat, step the right foot back, bending the left knee. Make sure your left knee never extends beyond your ankle. Turn your right toes out at a 45-degree angle. Bring your left forearm to your left thigh, using your hand to support your belly if you'd like. Reach the right arm over your ear, palm of the hand facing down. If it's comfortable for your neck look up, otherwise look down. Breathe into the right side body and lung, holding this posture for 2 to 3 breaths.

After the first breaths, begin to move the extended arm in a large circle to help bring movement and promote mobility and comfort in the shoulder. Imagine you are using a lasso or trying to make the biggest circle possible while keeping the movement fluid and smooth. Allow the head and neck to move naturally with the arm so that there is no straining in the neck. Take several circles in one direction before changing directions and repeating the pose on the other side.

18.   Utkata Konasana (Goddess Pose), *variation*

Standing from the top of your mat, step the right foot back. Take a wide stance with your feet, your toes turning out at 45-degree angles. You should be facing the right side of your mat. Bend your knees and take a low squat position. If you feel any pressure or pain in the pelvic area, bring your feet together and do not bend your knees as deep. Lift your front hipbones up as you lengthen your tailbone down towards the mat. Soften your front ribs so as to not exaggerate the sway in your low back.

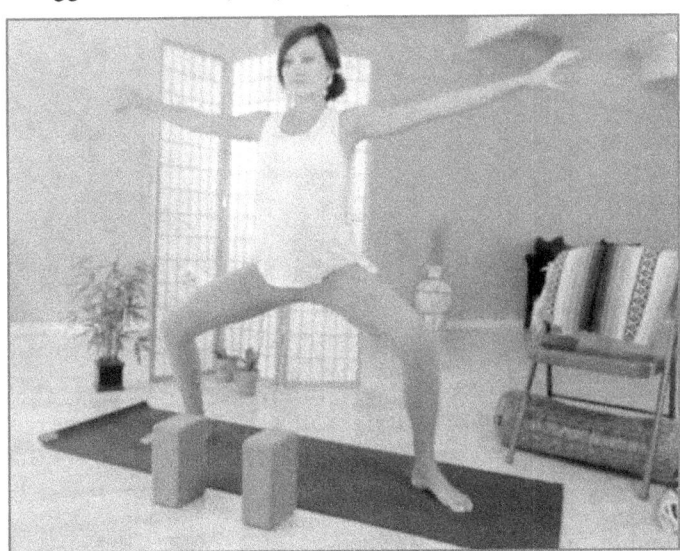

Take your arms out to your sides, bringing them level with the floor. Imagine as if you have a doorknob in each hand. Focusing on the breath, begin to turn the doorknobs back and forth. You can go as fast or as slow as is comfortable.

As simple as this exercise is, you should start to feel the muscles of the arms fatigue. Try not to compensate with the muscles of the neck – keep the neck relaxed and the throat and jaw soft.

This movement is great for strengthening the muscles necessary to maintain good posture (which means comfort) during the 9 months of pregnancy, as well as preparing the muscles for the workout they will receive once baby is born – rocking, breastfeeding, carrying car seat in and out, etc.

See if you can repeat this pose twice, taking a short break in between by lowering the arms and straightening the legs. The more your practice, the longer you should be able to hold this pose and work the arms.

19. Prasarita Padottanasana (Wide Legged Forward Bend)

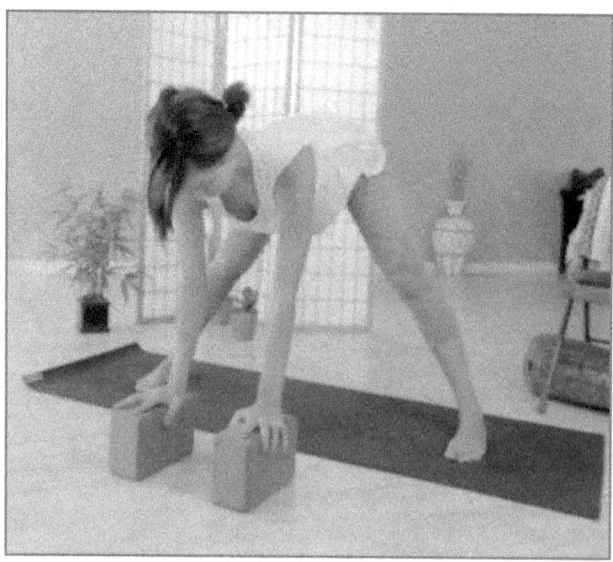

From the wide-legged stance in the pose above, straighten the legs, making sure your toes are pointing to the long edge of the mat and the sides of your feet are parallel with the short ends of your mat. Have two blocks in front of you or something that you can elevate your hands on.

Engage your quadriceps muscles by lifting the kneecaps up. Rotate the upper inner thighs back to create more space in your low back. Without compressing the belly at all, begin to hinge forward from your hips, placing your hands on the blocks when your tummy begins to touch your hip creases. (If you are in your 1st or 2nd trimester you may be able to go a bit deeper, possibly not needing the blocks so long as there is no compression in the abdomen. If you are further along in your 3rd trimester, keep your spine level with the ground, creating a hammock-type of position for your baby.)

To deepen the stretch, make sure your hips stay over your ankles and you are extending through the spine, keeping the heart and the chest open. Hold this pose for 5 to 6 breaths or as long as is comfortable. Be mindful as you exit the pose, as it is common to feel lightheaded or dizzy thanks to the elevated volume of blood that is running through the body.

20. Prasarita Padottanasana (Wide Legged Forward Bend), *variation*

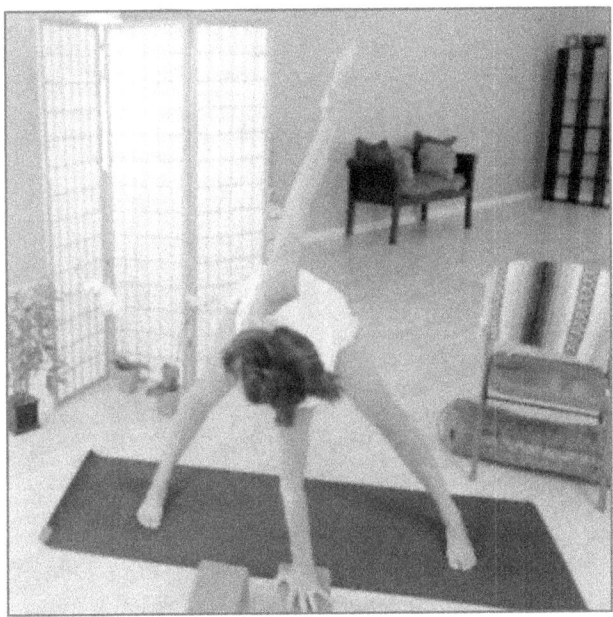

As a variation to the pose described above, you can add open twists, which feel great for the back and shoulders. While many twists should not be performed during pregnancy because of the compression and squeezing, this variation is safe and is a great alternative. From the modified Wide Legged Forward Bend, bring your left hand directly in front of your body on the block. With an inhalation, reach your right hand up towards the ceiling, initiating the twist from your ribs. If it is comfortable for your neck, bring your gaze up towards the top hand. As you exhale return both hands down the blocks or floor. With your next inhalation, twist to the other side – right hand down, left arm up.

Continue moving with the breath, repeating the twist at least 3 times on each side, before pausing in the center and slowly bringing yourself back up to stand. Again, be mindful as you bring yourself up, as it is normal to feel slightly dizzy or lightheaded after this exercise.

21. Ardha Chandrasana (Half Moon Pose)

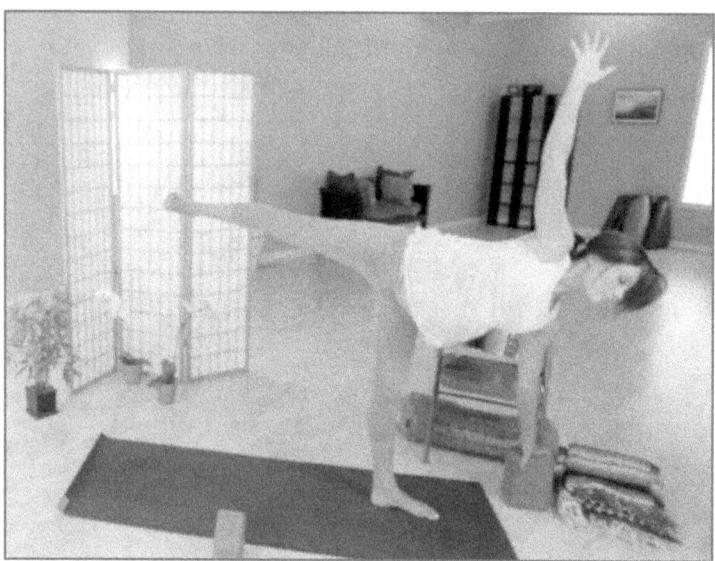

From a standing position at the top of your mat, step the right foot back. Have a block nearby on your left side. Bend your left knee, transferring your weight completely off the right leg. With your left hand on the block at your side, carefully begin to lift the right leg off the floor. Move the left hand so that stays directly under your shoulder. Engage the left leg by lifting the kneecap up. Continue to lift the right leg higher, possibly getting it level with the floor.

See if you can open your torso, turning the right ribs up towards the ceiling and bringing the right hip over the left. Flex your right foot and breathe deep into right side body. Hold this pose for 5 to 6 breaths before bending the left knee and carefully placing the right foot back to the floor. Repeat the pose on the other side.

It is very important to avoid falling when performing this posture. If this pose is new to you or you are feeling off balance, try doing Half Moon against a wall. The same steps described above will be used; only your entire back body will be up against the wall, providing support and stabilization.

22. **Utkatasana (Chair Pose),** *variation*

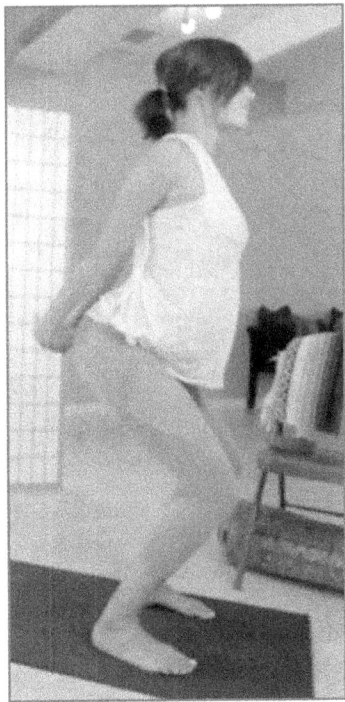

Stand at the top of your mat with your feet hip-width apart or slightly wider. Bend your knees as if you are sitting in an invisible chair behind you. Make sure your knees stay behind your toes. The further along you get in your pregnancy, the less you should be deep squatting in this position. Even just a slight bend in the knees can provide you with great strengthening for the legs.

Bring your hands behind your back and interlace your fingers. Press through the knuckles of your hands as you begin to reach them towards the ceiling. Make sure to keep your face, especially your jaw, relaxed as you work in this posture. Hold this position for 4 to 5 breaths before releasing the hands, changing the interlacing so that the opposite thumb is on top, and then repeating for another 4 to 5 breaths.

23. Utkatasana (Chair Pose), *variation*

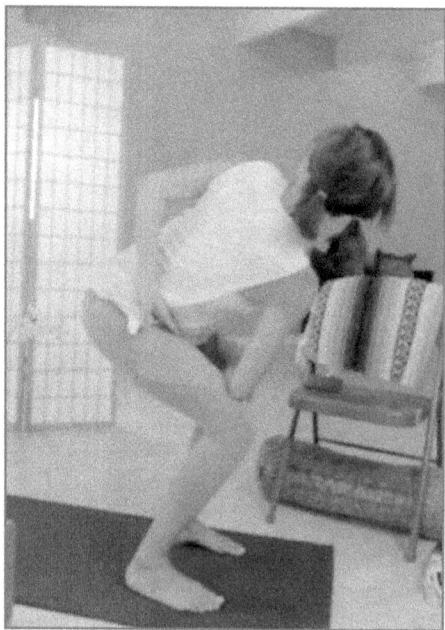

Stand at the top of your mat with your feet hip-width apart or wider, toes pointing straight forward. Bend your knees slightly, imagining you are sitting down in a chair behind you. As you bend your knees make sure they do not extend over your toes. Place your right elbow on your right thigh and your right hand on your left thigh, twisting the spine to the left. If you feel like there is too much compression on the belly, do not bend your knees as much.

Extend your left arm up towards the ceiling as you continue to draw your right ribs forward and your left ribs up. If you would like to intensify the stretch, bring your left hand behind your back, placing the fingers on the top of the right thigh. Hold this pose for 3 to 4 breaths before coming back to center and repeating on the other side.

24. Vrksasana (Tree Pose)

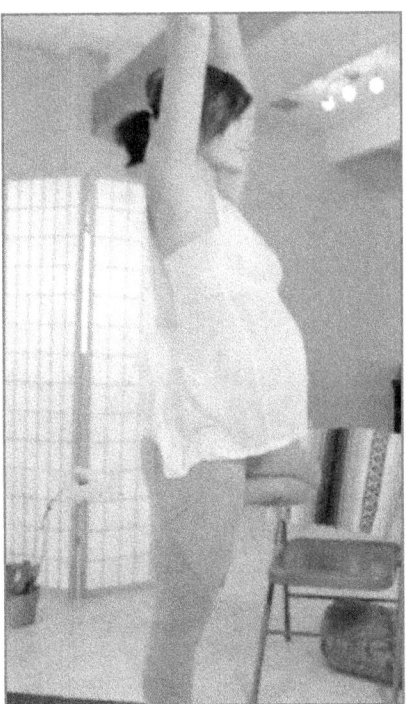

Begin by standing at the top of your mat. Engage your right leg, creating a strong pillar by lifting the kneecap up. Begin to shift your weight into the right foot, slowly lifting the left foot off the ground. You can bring the sole of the left foot to the right shin or calf or place it all the way on the right inner thigh. Be sure not to place the left foot on the right kneecap.

Press firmly through the sole of the left foot as you begin to take the left knee to the side, opening the hip. Lift your front hipbones up as you draw your tailbone down towards your heels. Keeping the front rib bones soft, extend the arms up over your head, palms facing each other and shoulders relaxed. Hold this pose for as long as you can or as long as is comfortable.

If balance has become increasingly difficult during your pregnancy, do not risk the chance of falling in this pose. Instead, use a chair to support the left leg, placing the sole of the foot on top of it.

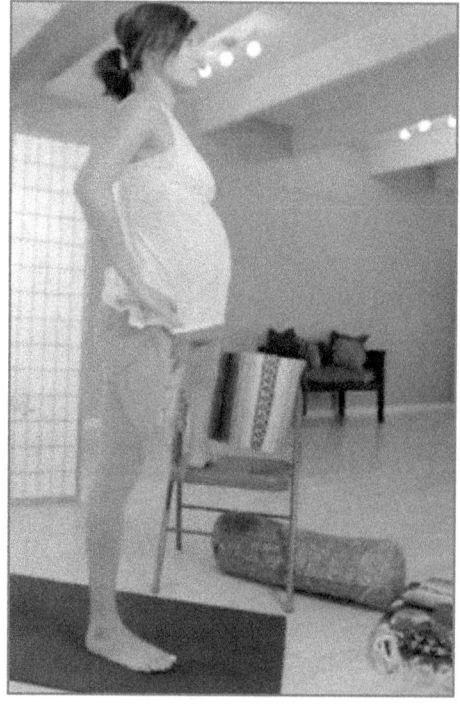

You will still take the knee to the side and find the same length in the spine and opening in the ribs, only you will be more supported – which means you will also be able to hold the pose longer and enjoy the benefits.

25. Standing Pelvic Circles

Begin by standing at the top of your mat with your feet hip-width apart or wider. Put a small bend in your knees so that you have freedom to move in your spine and hips. Place your hands on your hips and, as if you were hula hooping, begin to move your hips in a circle. Don't worry about what you look like – let go. Allow the movement to be fluid and smooth, focusing only on what it feels like. You can go as fast or as slow as you'd like, just remain mindful to the breath.

Go in one direction several times before changing directions. Perform this exercise for as long as feels good. Enjoy momma!

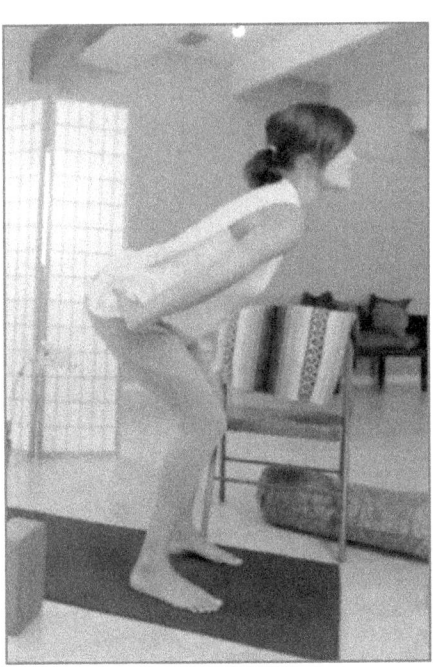
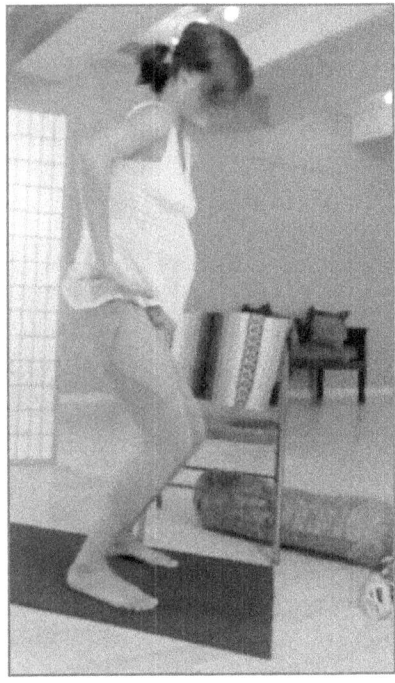

MOMMY DOES YOGA REST AND RESTORE POSES

Do these poses after your active practice or on their own on days when you need to rest and relax. Many of these poses can even be done in bed! Being restorative poses, there is no time limit to any of them. As long as they feel good, keep doing them! I promise, ten to fifteen minutes in a prenatal Savasana can change your entire day.

1. **Ardha Padmasana (Half Lotus), *variation***

   Take a seat on a chair, preferably one without much cushion. Make sure your feet can comfortably touch the floor. If they don't, place something under them, like a box. Lift your left foot off the floor and set the left ankle on top of the right thigh. Flex your left foot to keep the knee comfortable. Gently press your left hand into the left thigh, working to eventually get the left knee level with the right. Gently tip your pelvis forward, rocking your weight towards the front of your chair, to deepen the stretch. Keep the spine long and the heart lifted.

   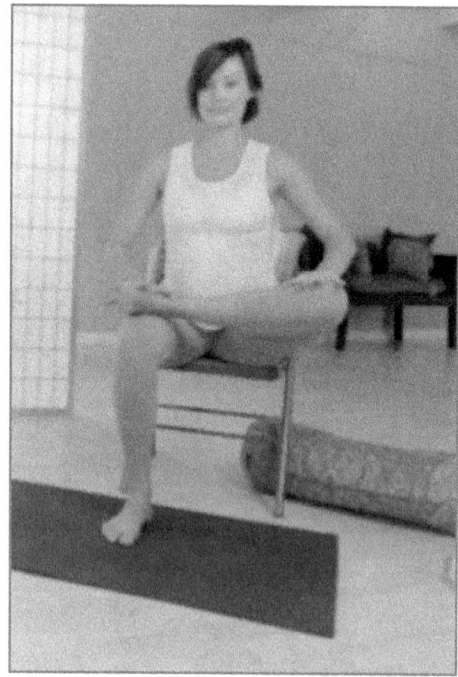

This pose is great for relieving discomfort and pain in the lower back, especially sciatica. Stay here as long as is comfortable before switching sides.

If you are not as far along or feel like you have enough room, you can perform this posture on the ground. On the ground, still elevate your hips, either with blankets or a thin bolster.

2. **Jaw And Temple Massage**

No matter where you are in your pregnancy, whether you are feeling wonderful with a ton of energy or nauseous and comatose, all pregnant women feel additional stress with the daily physical changes and emotional anticipation. This stress almost always manifests physically, and one of the most common places that it is stored is the jaw and face. Massaging the jawbone and temples on a daily basis can help relieve the tension that builds up and keep the rest of the body relaxed as well. Keeping the jaw relaxed, especially, can be very beneficial for labor and delivery as well, as those muscles translate to the muscles that are used for delivering with more ease, possibly even preventing the risk of tearing.

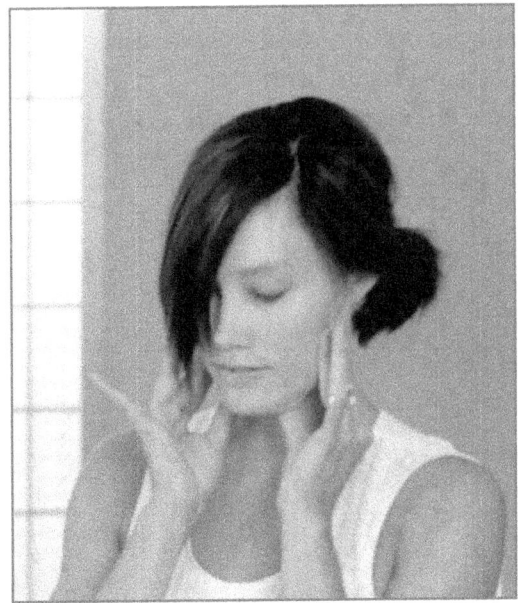

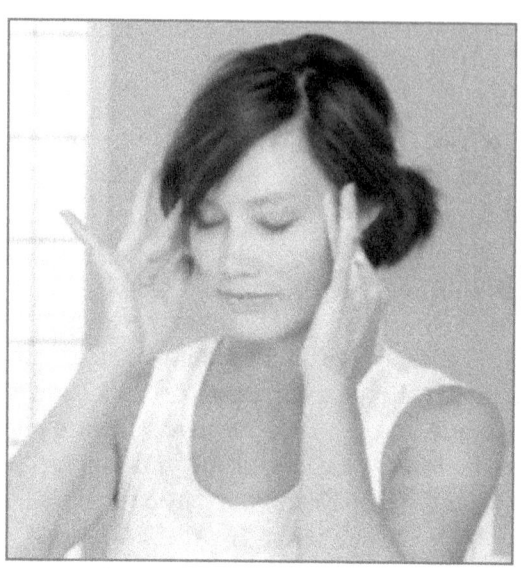

Take advantage of any spare time you have, even if it's just a few seconds like at a traffic light, to massage these two areas. Or add the massage to any of the restorative yoga poses listed in this section.

3. **Virasana (Hero's Pose),** *variation*

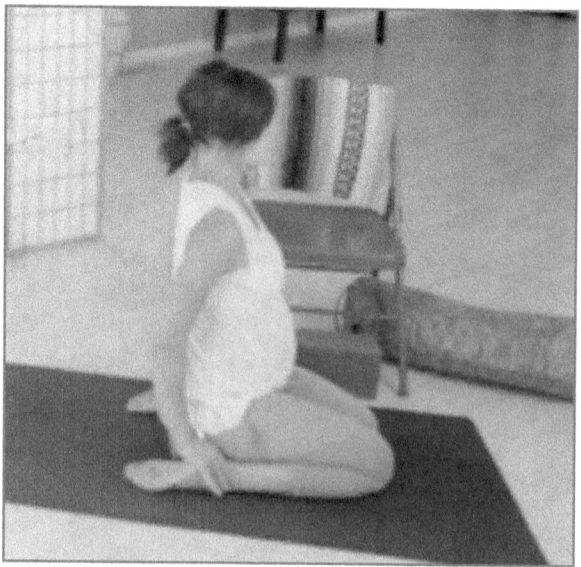

From all fours on your mat, bring your knees together while separating your feet wide enough so that you can set your hips between them. Use as many blocks or bolsters or cushions as necessary to sit comfortably, making sure your knees feel pleasant and there is plenty of room between the tummy and thighs. Your heels should be snug against your outer thighs with the tops of your feet on the floor. You should feel like you have lots of length in the spine in this position. If you don't, make sure your weight is evenly distributed through your pelvis and your spine is stacked naturally, including the neck. This pose is great for keeping the joints of your knees and ankles during pregnancy, reducing fluid retention that can result in swelling, as well as discomfort.

This posture lends itself well to adding various arm and shoulder stretches as well as strengthening exercises. Adding Gomukha *(Cow Face)* arms feels especially soothing.

Making sure right arm bone is drawn into the shoulder socket, extend your right arm up by your ear, palm facing your left side. Bend your right elbow and bring the palm of your right hand down the back of your neck and between your shoulder blades. You can either use your left hand to intensify the stretch by gently pressing on your right elbow, or you can bring your left hand behind your back, palm facing away from you, bending the elbow and reaching for the right fingertips. If you cannot reach your fingertips, you can use a strap (or something like it – dog leash, scarf, etc.) to bridge the gap.

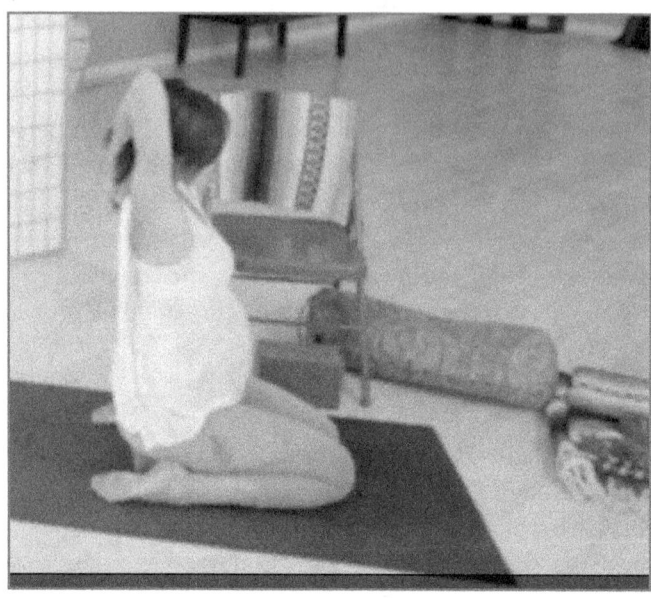

Hold this stretch for 5 to 10 breaths on one side before switching arms.

4. **Malasana (Garland Pose),** *variation*

   From a standing position, take your feet the width of the mat, toes pointing out at a 45-degree angle. Have 1 to 2 blocks behind you, stacked so that your entire pelvis will be supported. Bend your knees and come into a deep squat, resting on top of the blocks. Bring your elbows inside your legs, pressing them into your inner thighs. Join your palms together in prayer position. Lengthen the spine and breathe deeply. Stay here for as long as you would like.

   If you would like to get even more comfortable, do this pose against a wall so that your back is completely supported.

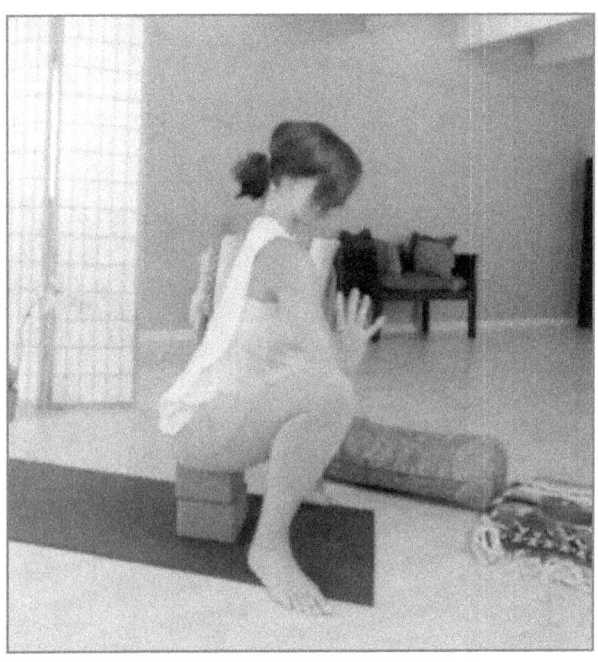

5. **Janu Sirsasana (Head To Knee Forward Bend),** *variation*

Fold two or more blankets, stacking them on top of each other in the center of your mat. Angle the blankets so that they are in a diamond position. Sit down on the edge of the blankets so that the tip of the diamond is in line with your pubic bone. Spread your legs wide, like a straddle. Bend your left knee and bring the sole of your foot to the upper thigh of the right leg. With a strap in hand, twist slightly towards your right leg. As your belly grows the less you will be able to twist, as it should not be compressed with the thigh.

Hook the strap over the sole of your right foot. Flex your foot and make sure the toes are pointing straight up towards the ceiling. Pull the ends of the strap with both hands, bending the elbows and leaning forward slightly – as much as you have space for. To intensify the stretch, rock your weight into the front of the pelvis slightly and lift the heart, lengthening through the spine. Hold this pose for 10 to 12 breaths before switching sides.

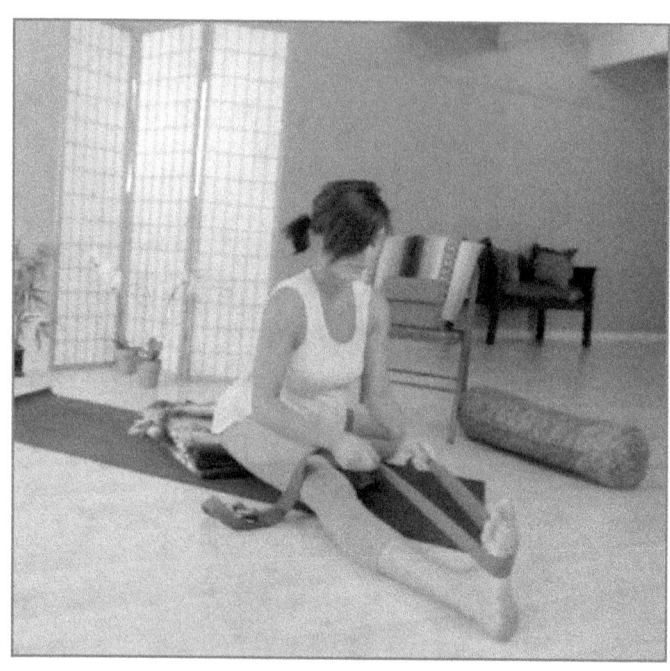

6. **Upavistha Konasana (Wide Angle Seated Forward Bend)**

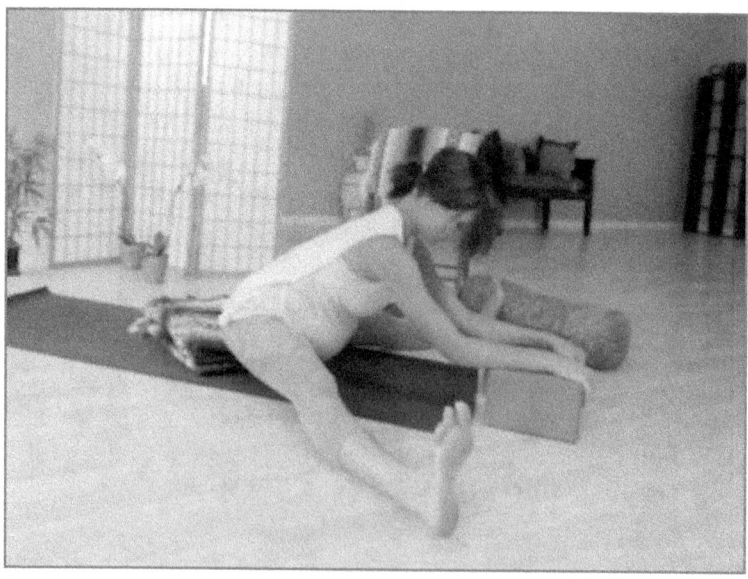

Still seated on your blankets as described above, open both legs back into a wide straddle. Flex your feet and ensure that your toes are pointing straight up towards the ceiling. Tip the pelvis forward as you begin to fold between the legs. Again, the size of your tummy as well as the flexibility of your hamstrings will dictate how far forward you go. Using something like blocks or a bolster to place your hands on can help create more space and provide a deeper sense of relaxation. Be sure to keep your spine long and the heart lifting, as this is key for keeping a deep stretch in the legs.

As you rest in this position, keep the back of the neck long by drawing the chin slightly towards the chest. Breathe deeply, thinking about elongating the spine with each inhalation and moving forward or deeper into the stretch with each exhalation. Stay in this pose for as long as is comfortable.

7. **Supta Baddha Konasana (Reclined Bound Angle Pose),** *variation*

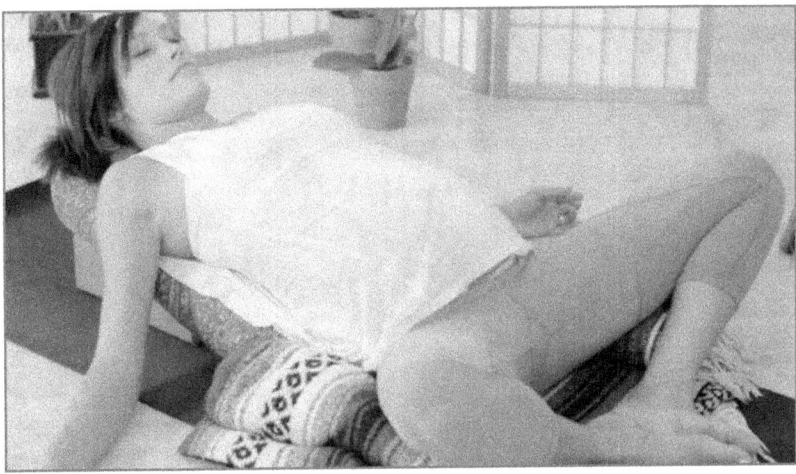

The supported version of this pose requires a bit of set-up, but is so worthwhile, and incredibly necessary, as your pregnancy progresses. For this pose you will need two blocks, a bolster, and at least 2 blankets.

Place your blocks, one in front of the other, on their lowest level under the top of your bolster. This should create a stable incline for the bolster, so that you are supported without lying flat on your back. Take your 2 blankets and roll them up tightly. Have the rolled blankets nearby, one on either side of you.

Sit down in front of the bolster. Slowly recline back on the bolster, bending your knees as you do. Once you are lying down, bring the soles of your feet together and allow the knees to open. Take your rolled blankets and slide them under your thighs so that your legs are completely supported in this position. Extra blankets can be used under the hands or arms or on top of the bolster if you need extra elevation.

This pose is incredibly soothing and relaxing, so don't rush out of it. Use this time to quiet the mind and connect with your baby. Focus on feeling the breath moving in and out of the body. When you are ready to exit the pose, use your hands on the outer thighs to help the knees back together. Sit up slowly, using your hands to help you up as much as possible.

8. **Prenatal Savasana (Prenatal Corpse Pose) – (Insert Prenatal Savasana Image)**

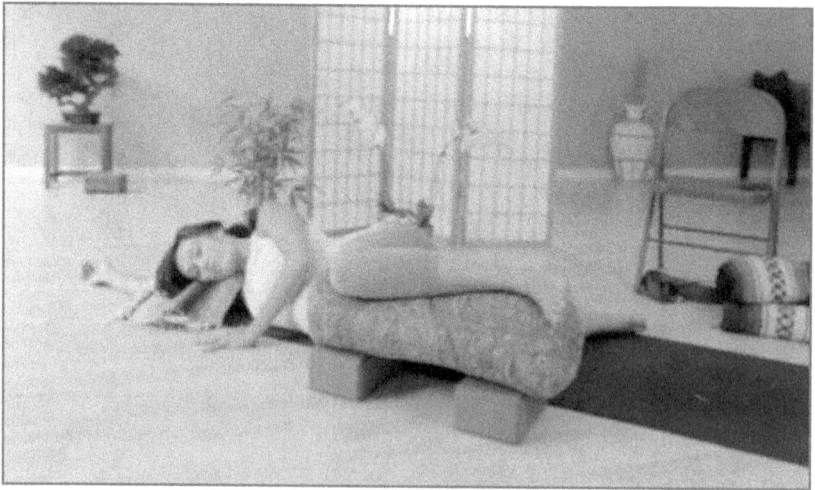

For this final restorative pose, you will want to have a blanket, 2 blocks, and a bolster. On either side of your mat, place your bolster on top of the 2 blocks, creating a sort of "tea table", with one block on each end. Have your blanket nearby.

Lie down on your side, placing your top leg on top of the bolster, bending it at the knee. The bolster should support the entire part of your leg from your knee down to your foot. You can either straighten your bottom leg or bend it slightly whichever is more comfortable. If you are feeling more discomfort or pressure specifically on one side of your body, particularly the low back, place the leg on that side on top of the bolster. Take your blanket and place it under your head and side of your neck. Your bottom arm should rest under the blanket under your head. Your top arm can be placed however feels comfortable.

Savasana, the final pose in all traditional yoga classes, should serve as a meditative rest. Allowing you to completely let go of tension in the body and meandering thoughts. Working from the crown of your head all the way down to the soles of your feet, make sure every muscle of your body is completely relaxed. Start by focusing on the breath, but as you rest in this pose even the thought of the breath should dissipate.

Stay here for as long as you can… and then stay 5 more minutes ☺

YOUR TOP 10 PRENATAL YOGA QUESTIONS ANSWERED

1. **When Should I Start Practicing Prenatal Yoga?**
   Some women wait to start doing prenatal yoga until they are far enough along that they have started showing or feel like their belly and changing body is beginning to impact some of the movements and poses done in a regular yoga class. But prenatal yoga can be practiced from the instant that you find out you are pregnant. There is no wrong time to start and there is absolutely nothing wrong with taking time to enjoy your pregnancy from the get-go. In fact, I have had women come to prenatal classes who aren't even pregnant – they simply enjoy the supported practice. Obviously for pregnancy, prenatal yoga can also be great for women hoping to get pregnant, post-partum, pre-menopause, menopause, post-menopause – it is fabulous for everyone!

2. **Is It Okay For Me To Still Take Regular Yoga Classes?**
   Absolutely. It is important, however, to make sure that the instructor knows that you are pregnant so that they can help you modify poses as needed and

support you when necessary. Most yoga instructors should be knowledgeable in caring for pregnant students, but some are not. If the instructor seems nervous about having you in class or admits that they don't know much about prenatal yoga it is up to you to decide whether to take the class or not. If you understand the basics of prenatal yoga (1. Create Space, 2. Don't Squish The Baby) and are in tune with your body, you can often do just fine in a yoga class, making modifications yourself and skipping poses that are unsafe or just don't feel good.

If you are new to yoga, however, it is wise to make sure you are in an actual prenatal class or with an instructor who is very knowledgeable. This will take any of the anxiety out of your practice and allow you to enjoy.

3. Will Yoga Help With Morning Sickness?

I say morning sickness, but know from experience that you are probably wishing it were only in the morning if you are one of the unfortunate to get it. The answer is yes. Yoga can definitely help with symptoms like nausea and vomiting. Certain poses, such as Balasana (Child's Pose) and supported Upavistha Konasana (Wide Angle Seated Forward Bend) and Baddha Konasana (Bound Angle Pose) can be great and, at the very least, make you comfortable as you rest. If you can find a time in your day when you feel less nauseous, even a fifteen minute practice can help curb sickness by getting the body and its systems moving and stretched.

4. How Does Prenatal Yoga Help Prepare Me For Labor And Delivery?

Prenatal yoga not only helps to strengthen and stretch the body in ways beneficial for delivery, but the emphasis on breathing and meditation can be of paramount importance when labor begins. Yoga can teach you to let go and to be present, two things that are crucial when delivering your little one. The idea of learning to be "comfortable while uncomfortable" is something else that can be taken from the practice – finding ease while challenged, stilling the mind amidst changes. Even simple yoga practices, such as relaxing the jaw and tongue as you practice, can translate into easier childbirth, as the muscles in those areas are connected to those used when delivering a baby. Not to mention that some of the movements done in yoga, like Cat Cow, for example, can help in the early stages of labor to position the baby and ease pain.

5. **Are There Any Types Of Yoga That Are Unsafe To Do While Pregnant?**

Most will agree that hot yoga should not be practiced while pregnant because of the dangers that are present when the body is heated too much. Although some women have practiced hot yoga throughout their pregnancy without any adverse effects or complications, I feel it is best to play it safe when it comes to the health of you and your baby.

Very vigorous or active practices, such as Ashtanga, should not be started while pregnant. For those who have practiced that particular style, one that is filled with lots of jumping and physicality, can continue so long as they are smart when it comes to modifying as necessary and changing their practice as their body changes.

Other yoga practices, particularly AcroYoga, should be avoided while pregnant because of the danger of falling and other potential risks that could be dangerous to themselves and their baby.

6. **Which Poses Should Definitely Not Be Practiced When Pregnant?**

This can be a difficult question to answer because it varies greatly from individual to individual as well as how far along one is in their pregnancy. As a rule of thumb, however, these types of poses should be avoided and are never included in a prenatal yoga class.

- Closed Twists – poses that compress the abdomen and squeeze and detoxify the internal organs (ex. Parivrtta Trikonasana (Revolved Triangle) and Marichyasana III (Marichi's Pose)).
- Extreme Core Work – poses that work the Rectus Abdominis or other superficial muscles of the core (ex. Navasana (Boat Pose)).
- Extreme Backbends – poses that overstretch the front of the body, especially the abdomen, which can possibly lead to the thinning of the lining of the uterus (ex. Urdhva Dhanurasana (Upward Facing Bow Pose)).
- Prone Poses – poses that are done lying on your stomach (ex. Salabhasana (Locust Pose)).
- Deep Forward Folds – poses that compress the abdomen (ex. Uttanasana (Standing Forward Bend) and Paschimottanasana

(Seated Forward Bend)).

* Supine Poses – poses that are done lying flat on your back, especially for an extended amount of time as your pregnancy progresses (ex. Savasana (Corpse Pose)).

7. **Why Is Meditation Important During Pregnancy?**

Meditation is one of the best ways to take time for your self while pregnant. It allows you to connect with your baby in an intimate and quiet way, helping to prepare you and your baby for the emotional, physical, and spiritual rollercoaster that comes with labor, delivery, and parenthood. Oftentimes people have the wrong perception of meditation, believing that in order to meditate all thoughts must be cleared from the mind. In truth, meditation is about creating a new relationship with your thoughts, shifting your perspective and learning how to observe, letting go as necessary. During pregnancy, as there are so many changes that take place with both mother and child each day, taking time to sit quietly and observe your thoughts can be one of the most powerful tools a mom has for learning to enjoy every step of the way, changing how she thinks about worries or fears, and adjusting to a new role.

And while most of the time meditation is depicted as a seated activity, it doesn't have to be if that doesn't work for you. You can meditate as you walk or hike or garden too. The important piece is taking time to be alone, to be quiet and free of distractions, and to tune in to all that is taking place within. As long as you are leading your awareness in rather than out, and doing so without judgment or clinging, you are meditating!

It's also good to remember that babies feel the emotions of their mother, sensing thoughts and attitudes in a way that can only be explained through the deep and interwoven relationship that is formed while growing in the womb. Meditation gives a woman a chance to be still and relax, to calm down when necessary, and to send positive thoughts to herself and baby. As with life, pregnancy is all about attitude and mindset, and there is no better time and place than in meditation to work on developing one that is positive, optimistic, and fearless.

8. **What Breathing Exercises Should I Practice For Labor And Which Ones Should I Avoid?**

The practice of yoga is rich with breathing exercises, part of a branch of yoga known as *Pranayama*. *Prana* means "life force" and *ayama* is translated from Sanskrit to mean, "control". Many of these breath practices can be incredibly beneficial during pregnancy, as they not only reduce stress but can help teach a woman about the importance of breathing during labor and delivery.

There are some exercises that should not be practice during pregnancy, however, including any that require the individual to retain breath for extended periods of time or those that use extreme contraction of the muscles of the abdomen.

If you are new to Pranayama, try these two exercises as described by Linda Spackman, a well-known yoga instructor and prenatal specialist based in Santa Fe, New Mexico. Spackman teaches classes at Yoga Source and is a director of the Yoga and Women's Health Programs with Surya Little at Prajna Yoga.

Basic Breath Awareness

- Allow the mind to be curious about the state of the breath.
- Bring awareness to quiet rhythmic movements of the inhalations and exhalations.
- Gradually lengthen exhalations.
- Allow inhalations to deepen as a result of longer exhalations.

Ujjayi – Upward Conquest Breath

- From basic breath awareness *(above)*, begin to "hear" the sound of the breath in the sinuses and back of throat. This deeper, sounded breath is *Ujjayi.*
- Alternate one *Ujjayi* breath with two normal breaths.
- This is one cycle of *Ujjayi.*
- Practice six to ten complete cycles.
- Rest in Savasana and observe the results of the practice.

9. Is It Really Unsafe For Me To Lay On My Back While Pregnant?

I don't know how many times I have heard, "Don't lie flat on your back!" or "Don't sleep on your back," during both of my pregnancies, especially in the yoga world. The reason behind this is that the weight of the baby can slow the flow of blood to your heart when you are positioned flat on your back, causing, in turn, a reduced flow of blood to your baby as well. And while potentially this could be harmful to a developing fetus (blood supplies nutrients and nutrients equate to proper growth and development) most doctors agree that if it is comfortable for a pregnant woman, a few minutes at a time won't put either mom or baby at risk.

The best advice I ever received was from a wonderful instructor of mine who told me that if my body is sending off warning signals everything is fine. And while she isn't a doctor, that piece of wisdom resonated with me. Our bodies, especially while pregnant, know what they are doing. They don't need us to tell them to grow our uterus, smash our bladder, or practice contractions – they do it on their own. If something isn't going right, there are signs they give us to alert us that they need help (think sharp pains, leaking of various fluids, reduced fetal activity, etc.). If lying on our back started to cause problems for the body, it should signal that something isn't right and you would innately know to change positions.

With all of that said, however, if there is potential risk to lying on your back it is best to avoid it when possible. Which is why in most prenatal yoga classes, for example, no time is ever spent lying flat on your back, especially as you progress into your third trimester and the baby is getting heavier. Does that mean that lying on your back for three minutes with your legs up the wall to reduce swelling is dangerous? Absolutely not. Most instructors, being aware of the risk, just won't ask you to do it on the slight chance that it could create some sort of problem.

So, again, the best advice is to listen to your body. If there is a way to be comfortable and do what you want/need to do without lying on your back then do that. If you need to lie on your back for whatever reason during pregnancy don't panic. Chances are you and baby are going to be just fine and, if for some reason something did start to go wrong, trust that your body will tell you and that you will be ready to listen.

10. Can I Still Practice Inversions While Pregnant?

Yes and no. Inversions can be absolutely wonderful during pregnancy. They are soothing for the nervous system and great for swelling and fluid retention. However, inversions should only be done by women who practiced them before getting pregnant and are very comfortable with their body in an upside-down position. The main concern about practicing inversions during pregnancy is the risk of falling. For someone who has never done an inversion, like a handstand or headstand before, falling is almost inevitable, which is why that individual should wait until after pregnancy before attempting them.

Even if you are very comfortable with inversions it's a good idea to take precautions when pregnant – like using a wall for extra support. You should also take into consideration two other things. First, how do you get into your inversion? If it is a graceful lift, without any jarring or jumping, then by all means go for it. If it is a fling-yourself-full-force-into-the-wall type of thing, then maybe it's not the best idea. Second, why are you doing inversions while pregnant? It's always a good idea to question your motive behind a pose, for everyone not just expecting mommas. If you are doing an inversion while pregnant for the oohs-and-ahs of others, then maybe you should reconsider. If your body is craving inversions and you feel amazing and light and free while in it, then you go momma!

Last point: Pregnancy is fleeting. Before you know it, you won't be pregnant anymore and there will be plenty of time for all the intensity you want. Enjoy your pregnancy and do what feels good, even if that is totally different than what you were used to or what you were expecting. You may not be throwing handstands while pregnant, but you are growing a human, and that is way cooler.

INDEX OF POSES

Sanskrit

- Adho Mukha Svanasana
- Anjaneyasana
- Ardha Chandrasana
- Ardha Padmasana
- Balasana
- Bitilasana
- Chaturanga Dandasana
- Janu Sirsasana
- Malasana
- Marjaryasana
- Prasarita Padottanasana
- Savasana
- Supta Baddha Konasana
- Tadasana with Urdhva Hastasana
- Upavistha Konasana
- Urdhva Mukha Svanasana
- Utkata Konasana
- Utkatasana
- Uttanasana
- Utthita Parsvakonasana
- Utthita Trikonasana
- Virabhadrasana II
- Virasana
- Vrksasana

English

- Cat Pose
- Chair Pose
- Child's Pose
- Corpse Pose
- Cow Pose
- Downward Facing Dog Pose
- Extended Side Angle Pose
- Extended Triangle Pose
- Flying Dog
- Four-Limbed Staff Pose
- Garland Pose
- Goddess Pose
- Half Lotus Pose
- Half Moon Pose
- Head To Knee Forward Bend
- Hero's Pose
- High Lunge
- Jaw Massage
- Low Lunge
- Mountain Pose with Upward Salute
- Plank Pose
- Reclined Bound Angle Pose
- Seated Spinal Circles
- Standing Forward Bend
- Standing Pelvic Circles
- Temple Massage
- Tree Pose
- Upward Facing Dog Pose
- Warrior II Pose
- Wide Angle Seated Forward Bend
- Wide Legged Forward Bend

Don't Forget To Stay In Touch At Mommy Does Yoga and Yoginiology!

Namaste

www.ingramcontent.com/pod-product-compliance
Lightning Source LLC
Chambersburg PA
CBHW060229290526
45789CB00003B/1470